CONTENTS

Title Page	
Notice of Rights	1
Introduction	2
Before the surgery	3
The day of the surgery	9
Day one after surgery	13
Day two after surgery	17
Day three after surgery	19
Day four after surgery	21
Day five after surgery, Day two at rehab	24
Day six after surgery, Day three at rehab	28
Day seven after surgery, Day four at rehab	30
Day eight after surgery, Day five at rehab	35
Day nine after surgery, Day six at rehab	42

Day 10 after surgery, Day seven at rehab	51
Day 11 after surgery, Day eight at rehab	55
Day 12 after surgery, Day nine at rehab, Day one at home	59
Day 13 after surgery, Day two at home	61
Day 14 after surgery, Day three at home	62
Day 15 after surgery, Day four at home	64
Day 17 after surgery, Day six at home	65
Day 18 after surgery, Day seven at home	67
Day 19 after surgery, Day eight at home	68
Day 20 after surgery, Day nine at home	71
Day 21 after surgery, Day 10 at home	73
Day 22 after surgery, Day 11 at home	75
Day 25 after surgery, Day 14 at home	76

Day 27 after surgery, Day 17 at home	77
Day 30 after surgery	78
Day 31 after surgery	80
Day 35 after surgery	82
Day 37 after surgery	83
Day 38 after surgery	84
Day 41 after surgery	85
Day 43 after surgery	86
Day 52 after surgery	87
Day 59 after surgery	88
Day 60 after surgery	89
Day 76 after surgery	90
Day 80 after surgery	91
Day 89 after surgery	92
Day 90 after surgery	93
Day 91 after surgery	95
Day 93 after surgery	96
Day 116 after surgery	97
Day 123 after surgery	99
Day 125 after surgery	101
Day 128 after surgery	104
Day 129 after surgery	105
Day 130 after surgery	107
Day 164 after surgery	109

Day 169 after surgery	111
Day 180 after surgery	112
Day 275 after surgery	114
Conclusion	115
Alphabetical Index	117

STEP BY STEP BACK SURGERY

A Recovery Guide:

What your doctor can't tell you.

By

Kady Dash

NOTICE OF RIGHTS

Copyright © 2017 by Kady Dash. All rights reserved.

No part of this publication may be reproduced, stored in a retrieval system, or transmitted in any form or by any means, electronic, mechanical, photocopying, recording, scanning, or otherwise, without the prior written permission of the author.

Limit of Liability/Disclaimer of Warranty: While the publisher and author have used their best efforts in preparing this book, they make no representations or warranties with respect to the accuracy or completeness of the contents of this book and specifically disclaim any implied warranties of merchantability or fitness for a particular purpose. No warranty may be created or extended by sales representatives or written sales materials. The advice and strategies contained herein may not be suitable for your situation. You should consult with a professional when appropriate. Neither the publisher nor the author shall be liable for any loss of profit or any other commercial damages, including but not limited to special, incidental, consequential, personal, or other damages.

INTRODUCTION

Despite my extensive research prior to the spinal fusion surgery, I had many surprises along the way, from hospital to rehab. Because of the privacy laws, my doctor was not able to connect me with other patients who underwent the same procedure. This difficulty in finding first-hand information was the inspiration for this book. There were a lot of things along the way that I wish I knew ahead of time. During my rehabilitation, I kept a diary to both keep myself busy and to help me recollect what happened and how I felt. This diary is the base for this book. I hope this book helps other people who might be going through the same experience.

BEFORE THE SURGERY

Getting ready for surgery and rehabilitation

My story of recovery from disk fusion surgery started a few weeks before the surgery was scheduled. I needed to plan ahead for several contingencies as I lived alone. I needed to prepare not only for what I needed to take to the hospital, but also for potentially being sent to a rehabilitation facility or coming back home with physical limitations such as not being able to walk up the stairs to my bedroom.

Researching rehabilitation facilities

Before going to the hospital, I scoped out several rehabilitation facilities so I would be able to tell the hospital where I wanted to be sent if I needed rehabilitation. I explained that I was about to have major surgery and might need a rehabilitation facility after it. I asked for a tour and checked if they had openings. I was glad that I visited the facilities as I saw that some facilities were nicer than others which was obvious in person but not from their web sites.

Packing

My tote bag contained a robe, a pair of slippers, a small fan, an MP3 player with an audiobook, and a paperback book. The only thing I used in the hospital was the fan. The fan was needed because the hospital rooms were very warm. I took a small fan with cloth blades, which turned out to be very useful because in the tight headquarters of the hospital everyone kept running into the fan blades but the cloth blades did not hurt.

I did not wear my own clothing because the hospital Johnny gowns were by far the most comfortable to wear as they opened in the back, and everyone had to look at my back.

In the hospital my mind was too scattered from pain meds to concentrate on the books (audio or written), so I was never tempted to listen or read.

I did not bring my cell phone as the hospital explicitly disallowed the patient's cell phones. The bedside phone was provided at no extra charge.

In this book, I will share a list of items I should have had with me but at the start of my journey I did not know these items even existed.

Preparing my home

At home, I reorganized my house so I could live downstairs for a brief period of time without going up the stairs to my bedroom and study. This meant that the bed, my clothing, my computer, the TV had to be set up on the first floor. Note that showers are not allowed after surgery for many weeks to avoid infections, so the fact that only my upstairs bathroom had a shower was not a problem.

The hospital and the rehabilitation checklists

The hospital provided a very helpful checklist of what to bring and what not to bring to the hospital. The rehabilitation place did not provide such a list. It was only after I got to the rehabilitation facility that I learned I did not have what they expected me to have. Some of the items they expected me to have were explicitly on the hospital's "do not bring" list!

Upgrading the hospital room

A typical hospital room has two beds. I heard it was possible to upgrade to a single room during the hospital stay. I called the hospital to find out if I could upgrade while I was already there based on the conditions, or if I needed to make this upgrade decision in advance. I was told that I could request an upgrade at any time during my stay, however, whether it would be possible would depend on the availability of a single room. They told me that upgrading the room is cheaper than reserving a single room (somewhat under $300 a day vs. slightly over $300, a hefty amount in either case). They told me to write down a credit card number on a piece of paper (the hospital requested that patients left credit cards at home) as the hospital charged for upgrade immediately upon the request.

Rehabilitation facility co-pay

I called both my insurance and the rehabilitation facility before my surgery to find out about the cost of the rehabilitation facility. They told me about the $500 co-pay, but no one mentioned to me that I would need to pay it prior to admission. The admissions staff requested the credit card while I was lying on a stretcher when they took me out of the ambulance! Since the hospital explicitly said I should not bring my credit cards to the hospital my plan was to ask a friend to bring my wallet with credit cards after I was situated in the rehabilitation facility. Good thing I had a slip of paper with my credit card number or I might have been sent back to the hospital. But I am getting ahead of myself...

Conflict between the hospital and the rehabilitation checklists

As a take away from this chapter I want to highlight the differences between what the hospital did not allow me to bring into the hospital and what the rehabilitation facility expected me to have with me.

The rehabilitation facility expected me to have a credit card before I was wheeled into the building. The hospital did not want to be responsible for lost credit cards and did not allow them.

In the rehabilitation facility, I was expected to have a cell phone otherwise I was charged for having a phone in my room, making calls, and receiving calls even if the calls were local. The hospital explicitly requested that the patients leave their cell phones at home.

THE DAY OF THE SURGERY

Admissions office

My surgery was scheduled for 11:00 am. The hospital instructions asked me to arrive 2 hours before the surgery. I allowed double the normal commute time (two hours) for downtown Boston traffic, but it was not enough! At 9 am we were not moving about three miles away from the hospital. I called the admissions office in a somewhat panicked state. The person on the other end was very friendly and comforting, "You still have two hours before surgery, just do the best you can. Don't worry."

Finally, we arrived at the hospital. The admissions area looked like a hotel lobby: cushy chairs, artwork on the walls, brass luggage racks, suitcases on the racks. My simple tote bag looked out of place!

And now you will get sleepy...

My name was called shortly after we arrived. The nurses told me that the surgery before my surgery went faster than scheduled and that my procedure will start earlier than planned. However, they wheeled me into the operating room at exactly 11:00 am, as scheduled.

Surprisingly, before the surgery I was very calm, my blood pressure and pulse confirm my absolute tranquility. Everyone was friendly and thorough. My name and procedure were verified at least half a dozen times by different people.

The anesthesiology team spent the most time with me, checking out my throat, my teeth, my crowns, telling me what to expect. They put in an IV flawlessly in one try – very much unlike a previous procedure I had in another facility where there were at least three IV attempts on both hands, and the IV site hurt for weeks after the procedure. The IVs from this surgery (I had one in each hand) left just a tiny dot, and no pain at all.
The last thing I remember hearing was "Now you will get sleepy..."

The next thing I remember...

The surgery lasted exactly four hours as predicted by my surgeon. The next thing I remember is "Kady, you are in the recovery room." I was in some amount of discomfort but the discomfort was tolerable. At that point the worst pain was a headache.

My next memory is the sound of strange singing in my room, a monotone voice repeating several discordant notes. It seemed to go on and on and my pain began to pulse along with the noise. I remember saying, "What is this noise? Can you make it stop?" In a short while the noise stopped and a woman appeared. She introduced herself as a Buddhist chaplain. She said that my roommate was a Buddhist and chanting helped her pain. She said she will stop to give me a chance to recover but will be back in a day. The thought of enduring these sounds again made me weak, worried, and upset.

The rest of the first day was uneventful. The pain was under control (I had a pain medication button which could be pressed to release medication every 20 minutes). I was lying in bed on my back, watching TV. The nurses were coming every now and then to give me various medications and to check my vital signs.

I did not need to worry about going to the bathroom because while I was under anesthesia, they put in a catheter, which was very comfortable. I never had a catheter before, so I did not know what to expect. I did not feel it at all. Bowel movement was not an issue because the pain medications cause constipation. In fact, it would take some work to get the plumbing working regularly again.

Because I reported a headache and slight nausea they put me on a clear diet: soup and saltines. Which was fine with me, I had no interest in food and was not hungry.

DAY ONE AFTER SURGERY

The worst thing about the hospital

The worst thing about the hospital was the noise level. Every doctor, every nurse, every visitor inside and outside the room, spoke at the top of their lungs. It is strange that the hospital does not have a culture of quiet voices, like a library. It would be so much better for the patients.

During the first night, I was woken up every three hours to check my vital signs. In addition, I was awoken by activity in the hallway, laughter at the nurse's station, doctor consultations for my roommate, nurses talking to my roommate while taking her vital signs and loud voices of the visitors who came to see my roommate. Everyone spoke loudly as if it was the middle of the day rather than the middle of the night when some people were sleeping.

My roommate was a very sick woman. A stream of different loud specialists continued to visit her all day, but at least this is the day the Buddhist chaplain gave me a break from chanting!

Physical Therapy session

In the afternoon, I received a visit from a physical therapy nurse. She told me that we were going to take a walk outside the room. After my first back surgery four years ago (a microdiscectomy), I was able to walk the next morning, so while I was lying down, I was under an illusion that this is going to be possible. After some serious effor, she was able to get me to swing my legs over and sit up in bed. I was in a lot of pain and no longer under any illusion that I would be taking a long walk. I was only able to make two small steps. These two steps took me to a chair near the bed. Going outside the room was out of the question. The back of the chair was at an angle that made me uncomfortable, and I took the two-step trek back to the bed. The exercise ended with me trying to lie down, which turned out to be more painful than sitting up. The pain was in my back where the incision was, and in the back of my leg, the site of the original pre-surgery pain.

You are going home

An hour after my two-step PT session, a care coordinator stopped by. She told me that I was doing well, and I should be ready to be released home in one to two days. Talk about mental stress: here I was barely able to make two small steps, and the coordinator told me that the hospital was ready to toss me out to be on my own in one to two days. I was in one of Boston's top facilities. Though the hospital was well run, this part of the process was not handled well. They should have told me that whether I was released home or to a rehabilitation facility would depend on how I was doing in a day or two.

I was stressed out and didn't want to see anyone. I made a couple of calls to people that said they wanted to visit me in the hospital and asked them not to come. Not having visitors relaxed me. I did not have to worry about how I look, what to say to make them worry less about how much pain I was in, or just having to make small talk. There was nothing they could do for me that the nurses were not doing. This was my first serious hospital stay. I had always been the one to visit people in the hospital, and it made me wonder if other people want visitors. My feelings about having visitors surprised me.

I asked to be moved

The next day loomed in my head as the day when the chanting will resume. I asked my nurse if I could move to another room because the sounds of chanting bothered me. The nurse said she would look into it. Later in the day, my bed began moving suddenly, and a few minutes later I was in a new room. This time my bed was near the window rather than next to the door. The room was cooler and felt more comfortable. Being near the window put me next to the air vent, and in this room, I did not need to run my fan. The window gave me extra light and a windowsill gave me an extra surface to put things on. This room was a real upgrade!

My new roommate was the most popular gal in Boston. She was my roommate for about 24 hours, and during this time there was hardly a moment when she was alone. Either someone was visiting her, examining her, or she was on the phone. Her bedside table was filled with flower arrangements, and the overflow flowers were on the floor. She had an unusual condition and in a teaching hospital that meant that a lot of residents came to examine her during the day and during the night shifts.

The second night in the hospital was again sleepless. Imagine how much more quickly patients would recover if they were awoken only for their own treatments.

DAY TWO AFTER SURGERY

I have grown fond of my catheter

I have grown fond of my catheter. Having a catheter meant I did not have to get up, which hurt. However, the nurse announced that she did not like something about my catheter and that it will be removed. She said if I needed to go to the bathroom, I would need to use a bedpan. I was not looking forward to this as lifting my butt hurts.

I was worried that removing the catheter was going to be unpleasant, but it was sort of like removing a tampon – you feel it slide out, but it was not unpleasant.

Bedside potty is not built for short people

By the time I had a need to pee a new nurse was on duty, and she did not want me to use a bedpan. She announced "We will be using a bedside potty". Using a bedside potty meant sitting up and walking, and I was not good at these two things yet.

Eventually "we" got to the potty but it turned out I was too short to use it. My feet did not touch the ground once I was sitting on the throne. When my feet were dangling in the air, I was not able to "perform." The nurse solved the problem by getting me a step stool. Now sitting on a potty was actually comfortable, better than sitting in the armchair next to my bed. I am 5'2". I am short but not unusually short, so I am surprised that the bedside potty could not be adjusted to fit me.

My third roommate

My popular roommate was sent home in the afternoon, and after about two hours, my third roommate was wheeled in. She was the best roommate of the three. She had a quiet voice, her visitors did not speak loudly, her doctors were loud, but they came in smaller groups. In a teaching hospital the number of doctors that visit each patient depends on how educational that patient's case is. I was visited only by my attending physicians. I was happy that I did not present any unusual or educational symptoms.

DAY THREE AFTER SURGERY

Sponge Bath

On my third day at the hospital, a nurse gave me a sponge bath. This seems like a small thing, but it made me feel much better. I was bathed while sitting on a chair in front of a sink. The sink was in the room rather than in the bathroom. The most interesting "tool" the nurse used was a shampoo hat.

This shampoo hat looked like a big shower hat, but it was full of warm suds. Once the cap was placed on my head, the nurse massaged my hair through the hat. When the hat was removed, the nurse dried my hair without rinsing it. This method cleaned my hair surprisingly well. Post-surgery instructions said that I was not allowed to take showers for two weeks to keep the incision dry (to avoid infections). I wish I had more of these shampoo hats, especially at the rehab facility! When I got home I was able to find them online. If I knew they existed, I would have taken them with me to the rehabilitation facility. No-Rinse Shampoo Cap is available on Amazon

Going to a rehabilitation facility

On my third day at the hospital, I was finally told that I would be released into a rehabilitation facility rather than sent straight home. The discharge was scheduled for Friday, the fourth day in the hospital.

Due to pain medications, I have not had a bowel movement in three days, which was beginning to worry the nurses. They gave me a bottle of Magnesium citrate in two doses (at 3 pm and 6 pm). It was supposed to have an effect about 18 hours later, in the morning.

In the meantime, I graduated to using the toilet, which was about eight steps away. The toilet was outfitted with the handlebars (which made the seat much thicker than a standard one). This extra high seat raised me enough that my feet could not reach the ground. However, the overall toilet height was lower than the bedside potty, so the step stool did not work as it put my knees very high, and that position hurt my back. I struggled with using the toilet a few times and then went back to using the bedside potty with a step stool.

DAY FOUR AFTER SURGERY

The last chores at the hospital

On the final day at the hospital the nurse's main concern was to make sure that I had a bowel movement before I left. Finally, in the late afternoon, the Magnesium Citrate worked, and the nurses relaxed.

The last chore at the hospital was to take the x-ray of the new hardware in my back. I asked to see the image, and I was surprised by long and skinny screws.

On day four I was moving better. I was still limited to just a few steps. Getting up and lying down was somewhat painful but I could definitely tell that there was an improvement. I could not twist my body, so I needed help wiping after a bowel movement. I could not twist my back to be able to do it on my own. Asking help was unpleasant, but the alternative was worse. There are aids to help people with limited mobility to wipe themselves, but the hospital didn't provide these. I will address my evaluation of several toilet aids later in the book. If I had known about them I would have brought one of these toilet aids in my hospital bag.

Overall, the level of pain after surgery, though significant, was considerably less than the pain I had after the actual disc herniation.

Moving to the rehabilitation facility

The ambulance took an hour and a half to make the trip that usually takes an hour. The driver picked the route through the back roads of the city rather than the highway, so the ride was very bumpy. I was hanging on to my stretcher to reduce how high I was lifted off the stretcher on every bump and slammed back down.

Abandoned at rehab

The ambulance arrived at the rehab facility at 1:45 pm. The admissions person asked me for my credit card, and then I was dropped off in my room. I did not see anyone until 6 pm. The last time I had my pain meds was around noon when I left the hospital. I was in pain, crabby and hungry.

When I was dropped off in the room, I noticed that the phone on my night table was disconnected. I asked why the phone was not connected as I wanted to make a phone call to let everyone know that I have arrived at the rehab facility. This was when they told me that the rehab charges for the phone and they do not allow even local calls until the patient pays for it. The hospital "do not bring list" contained cell phones, so I did not have my cell phone with me.

At 6 pm a friend (who guessed I must have arrived by now) and a nurse came into the room. I wondered if my friend's visit reminded the nurses that I was there. I told the nurse that I have been abandoned for hours and that I need my pain medication and some food. After the nurse brought me the pain meds and food, I began feeling better.

DAY FIVE AFTER SURGERY, DAY TWO AT REHAB

A new problematic roommate

My roommate at rehab was an elderly woman with a hairline fracture in her leg. She was uncomfortable and called for help every hour. The problem was the same as in the hospital, every person who came in to help her spoke very loudly. Despite having very good earplugs I was woken up every hour through the night. I have to say that the night aids were very patient and friendly and gave her very good care every time she called. I just wish they did not speak so loudly.

In the morning my blood pressure was 40 points higher than usual. I was very tired from lack of sleep.

My roommate had a stream of loud visitors. I was positioned near the door, so they had to see me as they passed by. Yet they spoke as if I was not there. Interestingly enough, they quieted down when someone visited me and then raised their voices again when my visitors left.

The room was very warm, and my little fan was fully deployed again. What a little lifesaver it turned out to be. You can locate this fan on Amazon, it is called Vornado Zippi Personal Fan.

Butt Buddy

During the first full day in the rehab, I had physical and occupational therapy. Physical therapy was walking with a walker. By the fifth day after surgery I was able to walk out of the room and make a short stroll in the hallway.

Occupational therapy introduced me to two very useful tools. As I mentioned earlier, twisting motion was limited and painful, and this meant wiping your own butt just did not work.

The occupational therapist introduces me to "Butt Buddy". This tool allows you to attach a piece of toilet paper to a long curved stick that lets you reach behind without twisting. If I knew about Butt Buddy in advance, I could have purchased it at a lower price on Amazon. However for expediency I asked a friend to buy the same thing at a local Medical Supply Store at whatever price they had, which was $64. Later on, I discovered that there is a better toilet tool than Butt Buddy, called Long Reach bathroom aid. It uses less paper, it is slimmer and provides a better swipe. And it is a steal for under $10 on Amazon, I bought a whole bunch of these as I was afraid it might be discontinued. Some Amazon reviewers are giving it bad reviews, but I don't understand why. I think it has a great design and worked very well for me.

The company that makes Bottom Buddy toilet aid no longer uses the cute name, but the shape of the product is still the same. My favorite toilet aid called is Long Reach toilet aid.

The second useful tool, but less critical for me, was "Sock buddy," which allows one to put on socks without having to bend forward. I needed to use this tool very briefly. That's why I do not put in the same category as a toilet wipe aid.

There are many versions of Sock Buddy sold on Amazon, some have a different names, but they look and function precisely as the tool I was provided in rehab.

Running a slight fever every night

In the afternoons my temperature rose to 100.4 degrees both days I have been in rehab. The doctor's instructions sent to the rehabilitation facility were to call the hospital if my temperature reaches 100.5 degrees. For anything below that the instructions were to take Tylenol. I was put on a Tylenol and remained on it for ten days. The nurses took my temperature only twice a day: early in the morning and just before bedtime. I wanted to monitor my temperature in the afternoon when my temperature began going up. I had a friend buy a thermometer for me so I could check the temperature whenever I wanted without the long delay it would take if I were to ask the nurse. This is another item I would add to the rehabilitation bag if I knew then what I know now.

DAY SIX AFTER SURGERY, DAY THREE AT REHAB

The second night at the rehab facility

The next night my neighbor had diarrhea that required her to call for a bedpan many times through the night. The staff was great – sympathetic and friendly. But they continued to speak in loud voices and never gave me more than one hour of continuous sleep.

My blood pressure continued to be 40 points above my normal level. I had a continuous headache. The back pain was under control with the pain meds. What I mean by "under control" is that I felt some pain, but it was tolerable.

The food at the rehab was slightly better than the food at the hospital. But I found it to be too salty. I was afraid to ask for no salt diet as I suspected it would lose any hope of having any flavor. Through my stay in the rehab facility the only times I had tasty meals were when friends brought me takeout.

DAY SEVEN AFTER SURGERY, DAY FOUR AT REHAB

The third night at rehab

The third night at rehab brought no diarrhea relief for my roommate and that meant no rest for me as well. After the third night of no sleep I asked one of the nurses if there were any empty beds so I can get some sleep during the night. She said "No" in a rather abrupt voice.

Luckily for me, an orderly overhead me and when the nurse left the room he told me that I should ask another nurse and gave me the name of the nurse to talk to. He told me that he knows of one empty bed and gave me the room number. Then another nurse walked into the room, and he whispered, "Ask her". When I repeated my request and mentioned the room number, the nurse thoughtfully said "No, this would not be a good bed for you. But there is another patient leaving today, I will see if we can move you into that bed."

In search of a new room

A few times a day I took a walk with my walker in the hallway for exercise. On one of my walks I ran into the admission person I met on my first day. When she asked me how I was doing, I told her that I have not slept in three nights because my roommate needed help with her diarrhea every hour. I mentioned that I heard that someone was leaving the rehab that day and wondered if I can move into that bed. The admission person said that the roommate in that room had something that might cause me to pick up an infection, so that room was not a good match for me. However, she said she would look into other options.

In the meantime, my roommate was taken off her catheter and every hour instead of nurses coming to her bed and helping her with a bedpan, they now wheel her past my bed, which is right next to the bathroom door, into the bathroom. Even the nurses began apologizing for these constant disturbances.

The new room

In the afternoon a nurse told me that I would be moved to a new room and to a window bed! The new room was much better, quieter, and more comfortable. Being next to the window also put me near a vent with fresh air and the temperature control. The new roommate was quiet (she watched the TV all day, which was a noise I found easy to ignore). She also had only a few visitors. By the evening my blood pressure dropped 20 points, by the morning after the first good night sleep in a week it dropped 20 more points back into the normal range.

Electric nerve stimulation unit – TENS

PT nurse offered me to try an electric nerve stimulation unit (TENS – which stands for Transcutaneous Electrical Nerve Stimulation.). After looking up reviews of it on the Internet I decided to try it. The claims are that it blocks your pain, but this claim is an exaggeration. The electrical stimulation merely distracts you from the pain. Once the unit stops the stimulation, the back pain returns after a very short time (minutes). The stimulation does not heal anything, but provides a small respite from the pain. Some insurances cover the purchase or the rental of the unit, and if you can get this respite as a covered expense – that is good. Otherwise, I don't think it is worth it.

Easy@Gome TENS unit is very similar to the one I got. Keep in mind that in addition to the unit itself there are additional costs of purchasing replacement pads. Each pad remains sticky only for a few applications, so they need to be replaced on a regular basis. For example, the pack of 16 pads for this unit costs $12.

One of my friends has a medical book "Lippincott's Quick reference book of medicine and surgery", by George Rahberger, 1926 edition that belonged to his grandfather, a doctor. I found it amusing that this medical book mentions the "Galvanic stimulation" for back pain, and it sounded very similar to the modern-day TENS unit.

Hair washing

Seven days after surgery I was still not allowed to get my incision wet. The "no showers regimen" was going to continue until I saw the surgeon for staple removal (two weeks and a few days after the surgery). I was doing okay with sponge bathing myself, however, the hair washing was a problem. Before the surgery, I cut my hair very short (great idea!), so I was able to get it wet with my hands, then put the foaming soap they had in the bathroom in my hair, massage and rinse it with just the wetness in my hands. I couldn't bend forward, so I could not pour water over my head because I was afraid to get water all over myself. All rinsing was done by running wet hands over my hair over and over again. Not very satisfying, but at least the hair did not look totally disgusting. I wished I had those shampoo hats the nurses used at the hospital.

As far as the kitchen is concerned I have not moved

As far as the kitchen was concerned, I have not moved. All my meals continued to be delivered to the old room, and then eventually made it to my new room. Needless to say the extra twenty-minute delay did nothing positive for the warmness of the food.

Curtains in the room

My new roommate was a perfect match for me. We were able to co-exist happily, and we both pronounced to the nurses that we were finally able to sleep well at night. Apparently, she had a noisy roommate before me as well.

I liked keeping the curtain in the room extended to ¾ of my bed, so I could not see my roommate and the people in the hallway, and they could not see me. My roommate never objected to this. However one of the nurses decided that she wanted the curtain open. When I objected she insisted. The total loss of control over even a few small things I thought I could control was very stressful.

DAY EIGHT AFTER SURGERY, DAY FIVE AT REHAB

Hunting Flies

The Rehab facility had a lot of flies. They were attracted to the light of the window and were beating against the glass near my bed. I used a magazine to swat the flies against the window. I probably killed six flies a day every day. I could tell I was getting better because swatting the flies became easier every day. It was a unique strengthening exercise!

Noisy visitor

My roommate had a visitor today. Why do people

speak so loudly when they visit someone in a semi-private room? I noticed that I had to hush my visitors as well. People seemed so unaware of the effect they were having on others.

A typical day

In my "normal" life I am a very busy person. I have a demanding (more than 40 hours a week) job and many hobbies that take all the free time I have. I rarely have time to veg out in front of the TV. Surprisingly, I was not bored at the rehab facility. Maybe being on pain meds mellowed me out but I did not feel any boredom. I found a few things to do. I typically woke up at 6:30 am. I would drag my bedside table to the bathroom so I can comfortably lay things out, I would take a sponge bath, wash my hair, and brush my teeth.

I like having breakfast soon after I woke up, so I would drink the tea I saved from dinner and eat a Newton bar (they were available in the nutrition room as a snack at any time). Then I would make notes about the previous day in my "recovery" diary. I would be done writing at about the same time as the official breakfast was delivered. I do not like eggs and sausages or pancakes for breakfast, so I would either skip most of the breakfast or ask for dry cereal. But I drank the coffee and asked for prune juice, which helped me stay regulated while taking pain pills. Drinking the prune juice for breakfast and dinner did it for me. Good thing I like the taste of prune juice as I drank a lot of it.

After breakfast, I went on an exercise walk with my walker. While walking, I was listening to my mp3 player with an audiobook. A good book made me really look forward to these walks. The corridors in the rehab were organized in a spoke formation. At the center was the nurse's station, and then four long hallways in four different directions. At the end of each the hallway there were chairs near the windows. I would walk each corridor, rest on the chairs and continue to the next corridor. I walked very slowly as moving slowly hurt less, so these walks would take a long time. But thanks to a great book, I was not bored.

After my walk, I typically had either a Physical Therapy session, or an Occupation Therapy session, or a TENS unit session. After the session, it was time for lunch. After lunch, I would take another long walk around the building. After the walk I would spend some time reading a book and watching TV. By the fifth day in rehab, I was spending more time sitting in a chair than lying in bed.

Dinner was served at 5 pm. After dinner I would go on another walk around the building. After a bit more sitting in the chair watching TV, my eyes would start closing, and I would start getting ready for bed. I would take another quick sponge bath, change into a new Johnny, and be off to sleep by about 9 pm.

Knowing what works for you

There are some things that the nurses might suggest that you might have to reject. For example, I was much more comfortable in my Johnny which I sometimes topped with my own robe. My incision goes through the waistband area, so wearing pants or panties rubbed against the area that was already rubbed raw by the bandages. Several times various nurses would look at me and ask, "Are you going to get dressed?" I would reply, "I am already dressed. This is what is comfortable for me."

I recall when my mother was in the same rehab facility for a leg injury she also wanted to stay in her Johnny but she was pressured to put on something else. She also said the nurses wanted her to wear a different outfit every day. I recall it bothered her, but she felt pressured to comply with their request. Once I gave them my firm response, there was no additional pressure. They could tell I was not going to be pressured to do something I did not want to do. My mother was too polite, and if she were firmer, they probably would have stopped pressuring her as well.

I also took every meal in my room rather than going to the cafeteria. Another complaint my mother had during her stay was that they pressured her to go to the dining room rather than eat in her room. I recall that they asked me if I wanted to eat in the dining room and my reply was a simple but firm 'no'. I did not have to explain. I really wanted to stay away from large crowds to avoid any possible infections. Plus everyone was about 30 years older than me on average, so I really did not feel like making small talk with people I did not have much in common with. It was much better to have a TV as my meal companion.

I think the nurses' attitude depends on how assertive and sure the patient is in their responses. They need to know that the choices are not out of depression.

Surprising differences between two wings of the rehab

My second room was located in a different wing of the rehab facility. This meant that the staff, the nurses and the personal attendants were different. The second wing of the rehab ran a lot smoother than the first. Things got done faster, clean up was quicker. The first wing had one nurse that was a bit abrupt with the patients. The nurses on the second side were all very sweet. Overall, the friendliness and helpfulness of the staff was very impressive. They were always smiling; they remembered everyone's names (even in the hallways) and recalled all special requests.

When I went on my exercise walks, I passed by my

old room and the nurses from the old wing. The nurses greeted me in a friendly manner and asked me how I was doing. They sounded genuinely pleased to hear that I was doing better and sleeping well. The only exception was the abrupt nurse who told me I could not move. When I said hello she did not respond. She appeared to hold a grudge that I asked to be moved. On the first morning after I moved when my breakfast was delivered to my original room by mistake, she tore up the sheet of paper where I marked my preferences for lunch and dinner. Another nurse had to piece it together with scotch tape. As I was looking at my scotch taped food choices in puzzlement the nurse who delivered my food explained to me why the paper was in pieces.

Tackling the stairs

On the eighth day after surgery the PT session tackled walking up and down the stairs. The idea of the exercise was to make the "good" leg do all the work of lifting and lowering. Since my pain was on the left side, the right leg had to go on the step first then lift the body and then I could put down the left leg. When going down the steps, the right leg goes down first. Surprisingly learning to walk the stairs again was quite difficult and painful. Going up was slightly easier. During the exercise, we were trying to simulate the steps I have at home, where the only rail is located on the left side. Going down I used a quad cane for stability. We also tried a crutch and a regular cane, neither of which felt comfortable. During the first attempt, I only was able to go up and down two or three steps.

If you need a quad cane to use on the steps, you need one with a small base (otherwise it does not fit on a step). My insurance covered both the quad cane and the walker fully. However, both items had to be purchased through a medical supply store contracted with the insurance. I could find the same items on Amazon at half the price, but the insurance told me they would not cover them unless I went through their supplier.

If you are looking for a good cane for the stairs, look for one the includes the words "small base" in the name Adjustable Quad Cane Small Base.

DAY NINE AFTER SURGERY, DAY SIX AT REHAB

My list of items to bring to the rehabilitation facility

After six days in the rehab, I wrote down a list of useful items. This list included items that I brought with me as well as the items I did not know about beforehand:

Earplugs and noise blocking earmuffs
Flent Quiet Contour earplugs are my favorite brand. They provide 33 decibels sound protection, and they are molded, so they fit my ear canal well.
I did not think of bringing noise reducing earmuffs to wear in addition to earplugs, but if I ever have to go to a hospital again, I will bring the noise reducing earmuffs as well because earplugs alone were not enough to suppress the noise.

Slippers
After back surgery, soft slippers do not feel comfortable. I found that Fleece lined Crocs were the most comfortable footwear because they are made out hard plastic with a very comfortable contoured sole.

Small Fan
Vornado Zippi is a small fan with cloth blades that I found it very helpful. The fan was always in the way, but bumping into the cloth blades didn't hurt. This fan is also completely silent.

Cell phone
Even though the hospital said not to bring the cell phone, if I had to do it over again, I would bring it and just keep it turned off while in the hospital.

Credit card
It is okay to bring the number on a piece of paper, and it is safer to have this information in case it is needed.

Long reach bathroom aid
Asking for help in the bathroom is very unpleasant, and no one can do it as well as yourself. I have tried several toilet aids. The Long reach wipe is my favorite.

Shampoo hats
These hats are great for washing hair when you are not allowed to shower. Later I found another option, which is a no-rinse shampoo. I think while in rehabilitation facility or right after the surgery, the

shampoo hats are better. I began using the no-rinse shampoo when I was at home. The no-rinse shampoo is more cost-effective, the shampoo hats are easier to use when your mobility is limited.

Digital thermometer

I used it to monitor my temperature on a more frequent basis than the official schedule. There are many good options. Any oral thermometer should be fine.

Supplemental food

This will vary from person to person. I wish I had breakfast bars with me. I was lucky that the rehab facility had Fig Newtons, which were similar to breakfast bars.

Notebook and pen

The notebook and pen were useful for making notes or keeping track of things.

MP3 player

My MP3 player had an audiobook. If you want to use an MP3 to listen to audiobooks, it should include the ability to bookmark so you can pick up listening where you left off. Not all MP3 players have this capability. I found the SanDisk Sansa Clip+ to work best for audiobooks.

Book to read

For variety, I liked having both a paper book and audiobook. I would listen to an audiobook while I walked and read a paper book while I was in my room.

Non-prescription medication
For example, I wish I brought my eye drops for dry eyes with me. The nurses got me some eye drops, but they were not my favorite kind, and they did not work as well.

26" grabber
I used a grabber to pick up things that fell on the floor, so I didn't have to ask someone for help. I own a large variety of grabbers, Unger makes the ones I like most. Unger grabbers give me such fine control that I was able to pick up things that I can't with other grabbers, such as sewing needles and pieces of paper. The grabbers come in different lengths. The 36" Unger grabber is the general-purpose grabber, however for the rehabilitation stay I found the 26" grabber most convenient because it was easy to bring with me due to its shorter length, and it was the right length to reach the floor from the bed.

Step stool
I used a step stool with the bedside potty and when sitting in an armchair as it gave me a more comfortable sitting position. I used a very simple and cheap Rubbermaid step stool.

Sock buddy
I used a sock buddy for a few weeks so I could put on socks without asking for help.

TV – a very nice setup

Televisions in the rehab facility were excellent. Each person had his or her own TV mounted on a very long arm. The arm was so long that I could position the TV to be anywhere on my half of the room. I could watch TV not only when I was in bed, but also from an armchair near the bed and even an armchair across from the bed. One of the attending nurses asked me if I wanted a TV remote. There were not enough remotes for every resident, but in a few days he brought me a remote, which made the TV even more convenient to use.

By contrast, the TV in the hospital room was mounted on the wall, and when the curtain around the bed are drawn the TV was covered by the curtain and not visible to the person in the bed. This meant you had to make a choice: you either got privacy or you got to watch the TV.

Handling nurses slow response

Needless to say, a good relationship with the nurses was very beneficial as they had information and access to a variety of things that could make life easier. I felt most of them went out of their way to make me comfortable, and I made sure always to thank them for small things they did.

When a patient needed something they pushed a button. The attending nurse typically would come within 15 minutes. The attending nurse helped with basic personal needs: adjusting the bed, providing towels, and so forth. The attending nurse could not dispense medicine. If the patient needed medicine or something else from the medical nurse, then the attending nurse passed the request to the medical nurse. It typically took an additional 40 to 45 minutes before the medical nurse would be able to respond to the patient's request. This meant that most of the time, I had to wait an hour before the medical nurse could provide what I needed.

Because of the long delays, I learned to plan my needs ahead of time. My needs were simple: towels and meds. I would ask for the towels before I needed them and put them aside for when I was ready to use them. Similarly, with the medication, I did not wait until the pain level was intolerable as I knew there would be another hour before a nurse could come to my room.

Assessment of my pain

Nine days after the surgery the incision pain was well- controlled with pain meds, which I took every 4-5 hours.

I still had a slight pain in the back of my butt and in the back of the leg along the sciatic nerve (i.e., the old pre-surgery pain). It was not as severe as before, yet I was hoping it would be completely gone right away. It will take a while before the continuous pain is completely gone, and I still get this pain if I walk for a long time six years after the surgery.

Nine days after the surgery I felt pain in the incision when I lifted anything heavier than one pound. For example, my back reacted even when I lifted a heavy dinner plate.

By the ninth day, it became easier to raise my hands over my head. Right after the surgery I noticed that it hurt to raise my hands to wash the hair on my head. By the ninth day raising my hands to my head felt normal.

The skin on my back was very irritated by the bandages. Even though they used paper bandages that are gentler on the skin, they were still irritating. The skin itched and was hot to the touch. The incision itself was doing fine. There was no oozing from it, however about half an inch from the incision I had a blister and a small hole. These two small wounds were oozing a bit. The nurses said these wounds were likely the result of removing the tape after the surgery.

The nurses decided to remove the large bandage from the incision to give my skin some rest. They left a small bandage on the two small wounds. I began applying aloe lotion to the irritated skin, and it began to feel better.

The first night without Tylenol

I had been running a slight fever since the day I had

surgery. The temperature rose every afternoon but less and less each day. On the ninth day after surgery, I had my first night without Tylenol and a temperature of 99.2 F.

DAY 10 AFTER SURGERY, DAY SEVEN AT REHAB

"Going home" workshop

I had been at the rehab facility for seven days. When I called my insurance prior to the surgery, they said I would most likely not need to go to the rehab because I was young, and if the doctor did recommend rehab, it would not be for more than seven days. Yet on the seventh day at the rehab no one mentioned a discharge date.

OT nurse told me that I am scheduled to participate in a "Going home" workshop. These workshops vary from week to week and the topic this week was nutrition for the elderly. "Eat more even when you are not hungry" was not a good match for me.

I saw that the previous "Going home workshops" covered topics like home safety, which seems more universally useful. The safety workshops recommended safety-related house modifications and various aids. I was hoping to hear about additional useful gadgets (similar to Butt Buddy), but they were not doing this type of workshop on the week I was going home. If I knew about these workshops in advance, I could have checked the schedule and joined the previous workshop that was a better match for my needs. My recommendation is to seek out this information early in your rehabilitation stay so you could have a choice.

When they solicited questions after the nutrition talk, I asked a few home safety questions. I asked about the best placement and orientation of the grab rails in the bathtub. I purchased a rail with suction cups but was not sure whether it should be horizontal, vertical, or on an angle. The workshop leader recommended two rails, one on the wall that is perpendicular to the side and one on the wall going across. My shower/tub geometry is such that I can only have one rail on the perpendicular wall. In that case, the nurse recommended using a vertical position. Through trial and error, I found that a bar on a 45-degree angle works best for me. Having a bar on suction cups is really beneficial because I was able to reposition it several times until I found an ideal angle.

Curtain Wars – Act 2

On that day lunch arrived with an attending nurse on a mission (the same nurse as in Curtain Wars – Act 1). "I will move the curtain open," she announced. It was not a question; her eyes were stern and unfriendly. I nodded: "OK, but I have irritated skin on my back from the bandages, and I need to lift my Johnny every 10 minutes to apply lotion." She stared at me. It did not occur to her that there might be a reason for needing privacy. "OK, I will not expose you." After this exchange she did not adjust my curtain anymore. The take away here: explain why you are doing something, it might help.

I was given a release date

At the end of the ninth day after surgery (seventh day at the rehabilitation facility) I am told that I will be going home in two days, on Saturday. This felt about right. The ninth day was the first day when I felt I could do everything on my own. I began moving short distances (from my bed to the bathroom) without a walker.

I was told that after my release I would have a visiting nurse come to my house to change my bandages, a PT nurse to do physical therapy, and an OT nurse to help me do things in the house without hurting myself. I was skeptical that I needed so many differ-

PT in preparation for going home

The last few PT session concentrated on the home environment. For example, we practiced getting up from a bed that did not have bed rails. It took some practice to do it in a way that did not hurt. The main useful trick was to swing the legs down and raise the body at the same time, so the movement of the legs helped to swing the body up without twisting it.

DAY 11 AFTER SURGERY, DAY EIGHT AT REHAB

Ordering rehab equipment for home

When my release date became known the PT nurse ordered a walker and a quad cane for me to take home. They arrived to my room a day later. Both items had problems.

The quad cane had a large base, which meant it was too large to use on stairs. The order should have been for a quad with a small base.

The walker I used at the rehab had nice soft handles, the walker that was delivered for me to take home had hard plastic handles which made my palms hurt after a five-minute test walk.

I said I wanted to exchange both items. The medical supply delivery guy was not too happy with me but returned with a new cane with a small base in about 10 minutes. He said that they had no other options for walkers. He wrote, "refused" on my order. He was about to leave when it occurred to me that I should check with my insurance to find out my options for a walker.

It turned out that my insurance would not allow me to order a new walker from Amazon. I was only allowed to buy medical equipment from a contracted medical supply store even if the price was significantly higher. They gave me a couple of names of medical supply stores in my area. I needed to call them to see if they have a different model of the walker. The delivery guy lost patience and said that I will need to return the walker on Monday (this was happening on Friday) if I don't want it and they will send someone to pick it up.

After he left, I started calling the medical supply stores. The two supply companies the insurance company gave me did not sell walkers. I called the insurance company again. They opened a research case for me, and towards the end of the day gave me the phone numbers for several more stores. It turned out all walkers had hard plastic handles, and no one carried a walker with neoprene handles similar to the one I have been using at the rehab facility.

After one day of using the walker, the palms of

my hands were as red as beets. A friend of mine had an idea of how to fix the problem. He made a run to the Home Depot and bought foam water pipe insulation. We trimmed it to fit the top of the walker, and the handles become much more comfortable.

The final bandage is off

My final bandage was removed on the 11th day after surgery. I have been using a skin lotion to treat the irritation, and the skin was feeling much better.

DAY 12 AFTER SURGERY, DAY NINE AT REHAB, DAY ONE AT HOME

Leftover medications

I was told that I would be given my leftover medications to take home. If I needed additional medicine after that I would need to contact my primary doctor for a new prescription. This all seemed okay, however, I neglected to ask how much pain medication they were giving me. I was thinking they know the dose of medicine I was on and they would know that I needed enough to last me until Monday when I could get a new prescription. However, they did not do any calculations like that and did not give me enough pills to last through Monday.

I should have requested a prescription to be written by the rehabilitation facility doctor, and I should have done it the day I was told my release date on Thursday. This way I could have picked up the meds on my way home from the rehabilitation facility.

Going home

The final paperwork did not take much time, after goodbyes and well wishes I was on my way home. The twenty-minute ride home was rather painful; I felt every small bump in the road as a jolt of pain.

After putting things away and settling at home, I was wiped out. I was in bed by 8 pm. I missed the hospital bed where I could raise the head and foot of the bed.

DAY 13 AFTER SURGERY, DAY TWO AT HOME

Visiting Nurse visit

On Sunday, the second day at home, a visiting nurse stopped by. We spent a lot of time on the paperwork, entering all my data into the computer, going over my symptoms, pain level, as well as reviewing all my medications.

DAY 14 AFTER SURGERY, DAY THREE AT HOME

Getting pain med refill

On Monday my main task was to get a refill of the pain medication from my primary doctor. The pain meds cannot be called in to the pharmacy, so I had to arrange for a friend to pick up the prescription from the doctor and then get the medication from the pharmacy. I had to figure out how to arrange for my friend to be able to get what I needed from my doctor and my pharmacy.

After multiple conversations with the doctor's office and pharmacy explaining my inability to be there in person, they told me to write a letter that my friend could present to them as an authorization to do this on my behalf. This took all day to organize and execute. I should have taken care of the prescription while I was in the rehab. Or better yet the rehabilitation facility should have given me enough medication to last a few days. The take away from my experience is to check that there is enough medication for a smooth transition to home care before you leave the rehabilitation facility.

DAY 15 AFTER SURGERY, DAY FOUR AT HOME

OT and PT nurses

On day four at home I was expecting visits from Occupational Therapy and Physical Therapy nurses. They turned out to be more useful than I expected. They gave me a few tips on how to do things. I have a lot of restrictions on movements (no bending, no twisting) and on lifting (I need to restrict the weight of items I can lift to 2-3 pounds). The nurses could have helped me to move things or arrange things in a more reachable fashion. However, I planned well, there was nothing they needed to do for me, but the fact that they could have done it if I needed help was comforting.

DAY 17 AFTER SURGERY, DAY SIX AT HOME

Staple removal

On day seventeen after surgery I was scheduled for a follow-up visit with the surgeon for staple removal. I also had to get another set of x-rays.

The ride into Boston was long and uncomfortable. I felt every bump in the road in my back. We had to make a couple of stops along the way, so I could get out and stand up for a few minutes as sitting for more than twenty minutes at a time was uncomfortable.

The staple removable was fairly painful, and I bled from the little holes. The staples were replaced with steri-strips. My incision was five inches long and was initially closed by 17 staples. Steri-strips are thin (one-eighth inch) adhesive strips, which are used to close wounds. They are applied across the incision, which pulls the skin on either side of the wound together.

The doctor said the steri-strips would fall off in two weeks by themselves. I will have to see him again in ten weeks. Until then I had to follow all the restrictions on movement and lifting. He said I could drive as soon as I was off pain medications and when sitting in the car was comfortable. The best news was that he gave me the green light to take regular showers starting the next day.

The ride back was even worse than the ride in because of the traffic. The return trip took slightly over three hours. By the time we got back, I was in a lot of pain.

DAY 18 AFTER SURGERY, DAY SEVEN AT HOME

After-effects of the long ride

The day after a long trip in the car I was in a lot more pain and more stiff.

All the three nurses (medical, OT and PC) came to visit because I was not available the day before due to the road trip. Each of the nurse's visits took about 45 minutes. They had a long list of questions that they needed to ask, checked my vitals, and watched me do some exercises. After looking at my incision they recommended holding off taking a shower for a few more days – the bottom part of the scar looked a little too red, they thought...

DAY 19 AFTER SURGERY, DAY EIGHT AT HOME

Better Butt Buddy

I received a new Butt Buddy bathroom aid. I decided to order a second one so I would have one in each bathroom. I ordered a much cheaper product ($10) figuring it will be good enough for the secondary bathroom. But it turned out to be a much better product than the Self Wipe product I paid $64 for, the one I bought from a medical supply store (which, by the way, is also available on Amazon for $27)!

The second tool is called "Long reach comfort wipe," and it has a rubber head rather than smooth plastic, which gives me better friction and better swipe. It has an excellent paper ejection mechanism, so you never have to get your hands dirty (the other aid sometimes needs fixing by hand). It uses less paper on each swipe and since it works better it requires fewer swipes. For some reason, it has mediocre reviews, but if you read the reviews carefully people buy it for different mobility limitations. Someone who has problems with their hands will have different needs than a person who has problems with their back. It addressed my limitations better than other tools.

Grabbers and Reachers

Grabbers are very important to me as I am not able to bend and pick up things from the floor or lean to get things out of the washer. I have a grabber on every floor including the basement, so I am not tempted to bend for lack of a grabber.

The best grabber for lifting small objects – including coins, sewing needles, and small pieces of paper – is Unger 36" Grabber I bought at Home Depot for $20. I have two of these grabbers because they are really the best I found. The 36" long one is great for the majority of tasks but they are too long for a few tasks (like removing things from the washing machine) . The Home Depot had only one length, however Amazon has a variety of lengths include a 26" Unger Grabber.

The worst grabber I have is the folding grabber with

suction cups. It does not close its jaws well, so it cannot pick up much, and it cannot hold anything for more than a few seconds. The only thing it is good for is picking up shoes – something that is not too heavy yet big so this thing can get a hold of it. Stay away from them; they don't work well.

My "laundry" grabber is 26" Dura-med grabber. It is not as good as Unger Grabber for picking up small objects. But its length and squeeze mechanism work best for removing items from the depth of the washing machine (one item at a time).

DAY 20 AFTER SURGERY, DAY NINE AT HOME

Assessment of my pain

On Day 20 the pain was tolerable, and I was able to reduce my medication to once every 12 hours. I still had incision pain, especially if I moved faster than a snail. However I also noticed that moving and shifting in bed was easier.

The pain became more intense if I stayed in one position too long (for example, sitting for 20 minutes) or walking longer than 10 minutes without sitting down.

When I walked, I still had a slight pain along the sciatic nerve (down the butt into my calf). I also developed a new pain in my big toe. The toe pain was a continuous dull pain. I was not sure if it was related to the surgery, but I did not have the toe pain before.

When I walked, I had to take small steps, and I moved very stiffly. The pain was less when the movements were small. I could lift two-pound items without pain (this is an improvement), heavier things still caused a reaction in my back.

DAY 21 AFTER SURGERY, DAY 10 AT HOME

Attempt to take out the rollator

When I walked outside I got tired pretty quickly (5-10 minutes), I have to plan my walk from my front steps to a bench in the yard and back. It would have been nice to have my rollator with me so I can sit down for a short rest anywhere. However, the rollator's weight was 10 pounds, and both PT and OT nurse wanted to see me take it out in front of them so they can make sure I can do it safely. The challenging part was getting it down the front steps.

I was ready to try it. Turned out I could not comfortably do it. I felt the pain in the back trying to shimmy it up and down the steps. Ten pounds was just too heavy for me at that moment.

First Shower

My incision no longer looked red and the PT nurse Okayed taking a real shower. The nurse stayed downstairs while I took a shower. This way if somehow I was stuck in an awkward position, I could yell for help. I did not think I would need help, but she thought it was safer that way. It was not a totally satisfying shower since I could not bend or twist to do the washing the way I would have done it before surgery. While drying out, I had to carefully pat the incision dry so I would not hasten the removal of the steri-strip stitches.

DAY 22 AFTER SURGERY, DAY 11 AT HOME

Three weeks since surgery

At three weeks after surgery I felt reasonably well. I was not in a lot of pain and was able to reduce the pain meds to twice a day or less. I still had pain at the incision site and in my calf when I stayed in one position too long. The pain in the big toe had stopped. I was able to walk about 10 minutes without resting. Overall my muscle tone was still in pretty bad shape because I could not do sustained exercise.

Three weeks marked the final visit from the OT nurse. The physical therapy nurse and the medical nurse continued to visit for one more week. During the last OT visit we practiced safe entry and exit from the car.

DAY 25 AFTER SURGERY, DAY 14 AT HOME

A setback?

I have been slowly reducing the amount of pain meds and stopped taking them altogether two days ago. I felt good for a day, but in a day the pain increased somewhat. The pain is in the incision as well as along the sciatic nerve. I could not think of any activity that was out of the ordinary to cause the pain.

DAY 27 AFTER SURGERY, DAY 17 AT HOME

Setback continues

For the last few days I was at a higher level of pain and resumed taking the pain meds. The pills made me feel sleepy in the middle of the day. Usually a one-hour nap fixed the sleepiness, but I did not like napping, and I wanted to get off the medication as soon as possible.

I was hoping to return back to work next week (one month after surgery). I postponed making the decision to later in the week.

DAY 30 AFTER SURGERY

Celebrex

Before my surgery, I used Celebrex to effectively control the pain. It occurred to me that it might be able to help me again instead of using the pain pills with their sleepiness side effect.

One of the very helpful things I did before my surgery was to ask the surgeon for his e-mail address. I asked him a couple of questions before the surgery, and he promptly responded. So I e-mailed him again to ask if I could try Celebrex for pain so I could stop taking the pain meds, as it would make my return to work easier. He replied in a couple of hours, saying that if I was on it before without problems, I could resume taking Celebrex.

I stopped taking the pain medication and took the first Celebrex pill a day ago. The next day I was feeling better – not sleepy and not in pain.

Steri-strips are off

Yesterday the last of steri-strips came off. One of the drawbacks in the construction of the steri-strips is that they are paper-based. This means their durability can be compromised if they get wet. I had to wait twenty days after the surgery to take a full real shower. After that shower steri-strips began falling off one at a time and yesterday I said good-bye to the last of them.

DAY 31 AFTER SURGERY

Prune juice, pain medications, and constipation

Pain medications cause constipation. There are various options for laxatives to counteract their effect. I found what worked best for me was plain prune juice. When I was on a higher dose of pain meds, I would drink a 4 oz glass of prune juice twice a day, with breakfast and dinner. Once I reduced the amount of pain meds, I reduce the prune juice to once a day.

For the body to function properly two things must be right: adequate water for absorption and adequate lubrication of the colon lining. Humans require eight 8-ounces glasses of water daily. This amount of water can be obtained by drinking any beverage that contains water, including plain water, tea, coffee, milk, fruit juices, soft drinks, or other beverages. However, milk products may be particularly gassy, due to the fermentation of milk sugar, i.e., lactose, in the colon. Also, note that caffeine is a diuretic which causes the body to eliminate extra water via urine, and this results in less water being available to contribute to lubricating the colon.

To lubricate the passage, the colon manufactures mucous. If the colon is dry, i.e., one has too little mucous as one does not drink enough water, the stool will be hard and dry and will stick to the colon requiring a person to strain to eliminate.

The dietary fiber (think of fiber as millions of tiny water-attracting particles) mixes with the stool. Each fiber particle soaks up available liquid and enlarges it into a tiny gel bead. These particles give the stool shape and moisture, making it easy for the colon to move along easily.

How does prune juice work? Prune juice supplies simple sugars that help draw fluids to the intestines. This helps to soften the stools, generate lubricating mucous and facilitates bowel movements.

DAY 35 AFTER SURGERY

Short-term disability

There were less day-to-day changes in my back. I had been off pain medication and on Celebrex for a week. The pain was there but tolerable; however, I was still limited to ten minutes walking without rest and about twenty minutes sitting without getting up.

I've begun working a few hours a day catching up on emails and doing some small tasks. During my surgery and recovery, I was on a short-term disability. HR department required official paperwork from the doctor documenting my "safe" return to work so until the paperwork arrived I was not officially working but it will be nice to start without a 35-day backlog of emails.

DAY 37 AFTER SURGERY

Hair Loss

From the time of surgery to about a few days ago I saw that when I was washing my hair, there was a significant amount of hair in the drain. Over the last few days, I noticed that there is less hair in the drain. I read that higher than normal hair loss can be caused by stress from surgery or illness as well as by some medication. I stopped taking pain medicine, and I am feeling better, so this seems to correlate to the hair loss.

DAY 38 AFTER SURGERY

Released by Visiting Nurses

Yesterday I was released from the Visiting Nurse program. The nurse wanted to have one more week of visits, but I told her I did not think it was necessary. I did not feel I was getting much benefit from the visits any more. It was helpful in the beginning, but the last week or two was just taking my vitals and telling me that I was doing fine.

DAY 41 AFTER SURGERY

Back to work

I went back to work in the middle of last week. I am working from home and part-time. I wanted to start with four hours a day, but so far it has been closer to seven hours. Still, that is a few hours less than my pre-surgery workday.

The main difference is that I feel less pressure and have been able to take several 20-minute walks throughout the day spreading out my working hours through a longer period. My goal was to walk at least one hour a day. My stride was getting closer to normal, not the tiny little steps I was taking right after surgery. However, the level of pain varied from day to day. Some days were worse than others but not bad enough to start pain medication again.

DAY 43 AFTER SURGERY

Going for a ride

My car has not been driven since my surgery; I started it a couple of times just idling but did not drive. I decided to take a short drive this afternoon to see how it felt. My town's library is about a mile and a half from my house, so that felt like the right distance. The drive took about 6 minutes. I was not totally comfortable but it was OK. Reaching for things was a bit uncomfortable, but I could anticipate the bumps better than when I was a passenger, and I could take more effort to avoid them.

DAY 52 AFTER SURGERY

Low tire pressure problem

Once a week I started my car and idled it for a few minutes. I noticed that "low tire pressure" indicator came on. However, trying to bend down to reach the tire nozzle with an air pump turned out to be impossible for me – too much bending, I just could not do it. So frustrating!

In general, I had to figure out new ways to do various chores that allow me to reach things without bending and twisting. I also had to learn and accept that for some things I need to ask for assistance. The number of things that fell into that category decreased as time went on, but I still have limitations several years after surgery and each person will need to learn what those limitations are.

DAY 59 AFTER SURGERY

UP the hill

I have been able to walk for 30 minutes without a stop for a few days now. Today I decided to extend my walk by walking up a small hill. It took me about seven minutes to get to the high point. I was pretty tired by the time I got there, but luckily it had a place I could sit and rest before heading back down. It was a nice way to raise the strenuousness of my walk.

DAY 60 AFTER SURGERY

Shopping trip

Yesterday I took my second car ride, back to the library to return the books. I felt more comfortable in the car than the last time. After the library, since it felt fine, I decided to extend the trip to the grocery store. It was so nice to be able to go by myself to the store of my choice rather than just tagging along with a friend. I meandered around the store with a shopping cart for about 30 minutes. I can't remember the last time I was shopping with a shopping cart – before the surgery, I had to have my rollator with me so I could sit when the pain started.

It was a good day!

DAY 76 AFTER SURGERY

Off Celebrex

Over the last few weeks, I have reduced Celebrex from every day to four times a week (basically every other day). Five days ago I stopped taking it altogether. There was a small increase in pain, but tolerable. From past experience, I knew that Celebrex continues to work for about three days after the last dose. Before the surgery, I could not stop taking it for more than three days.

DAY 80 AFTER SURGERY

First haircut

The last haircut I had was about ten days before the surgery, so it has been about 90 days since I cut my hair. I had the same hairdresser for many years, and she told me that my hair felt very brittle and it looked like I lost about ¼ of the hair I had before surgery. She told me that the good news was that she often saw hair loss after surgery and it typically takes about six months without medication for the hair to get back to normal. Her prediction turned out about right.

DAY 89 AFTER SURGERY

Going to the movies

Going to the movies presented a challenge, as it required sitting for a period longer than I can do without having to stand up. The solution was to sit in the last row, where I can get up several times during the movie.

DAY 90 AFTER SURGERY

Overall assessment of pain

90 days after surgery I felt definitely better then before surgery, however, I did not feel "normal" pre-back injury self.

Before surgery, I had no back pain, only pain in the leg along the sciatic nerve. 90 days after surgery I had two kinds of pain. The first was a pain in the back where the surgery was. The back pain started when I walked or stood for longer than 20-30 minutes. It also appeared if I tried to do anything mildly strenuous, for example, vacuuming.

The second pain was numbness/tightness in the back of my leg and around the ankle (the same location as before surgery). This pain started when I sat too long without getting up (more than 20 minutes). If I continued to sit the numbness/tightness became more intense.

Neither pain was as bad as before surgery. However, the pain was unpleasant enough that it took the joy out of whatever I was doing.

Frankly, I expected to feel better three months after the surgery. However, the people who had the same surgery told me that they were continuing to get better for a year after surgery.

DAY 91 AFTER SURGERY

Toro Power Shovel

After two significant snowstorms, I decided I needed an electric power shovel. I read the reviews of Toro Power Shovel, and it sounded like just the thing I needed. The product description said its weight is 12.5 pounds. It was manageable and was easier than lifting the snow with a regular manual shovel; however, it did not work well on wet snow, which is the hardest to handle.

DAY 93 AFTER SURGERY

Three months doctor visit

Today I had a three months follow-up visit with the surgeon. The visit started with an x-ray. The doctor did not examine me, just studied the x-ray. I described the pain I had and what activities caused it. The doctor said that I was within the normal range of symptoms. I asked him for how long I would feel changes/improvements. He said for nine months after surgery.

He prescribed physical therapy three times a week for eight weeks. PT should build up my muscles and help relieve the pain.

DAY 116 AFTER SURGERY

Physical Therapy – Isometric Abdominal

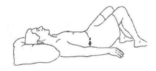

I started physical therapy. So far I had an evaluation and was given one exercise. The first exercise was trunk stability isomeric abdominal, and it should be repeated once an hour (or more often) sitting, walking, lying. I needed to repeat it every hour no matter what I was doing. The exercise was tightening of the abdominal muscles (as if you were holding in your belly to appear slimmer). The tightening of the muscles should be held as long as possible (until you are tired the therapist said), and the breathing should continue normally.

Even though this exercise can be done standing and sitting, the most effective version of this exercise is performed lying down.

Lie on your back with your knees bent, tighten stomach muscles by pressing your elbows down. Hold the tightness for 5 to 30 seconds at first, work up to 60 seconds when you can. Repeat every hour throughout the day.

In a study done by physiotherapists in Australia, the researchers concluded that people who suffered from chronic lower back pain could not efficiently contract and work their stomach and abdominal muscles. To increase the support for the lower back, you must retrain your stomach and abdominal muscle to work more efficiently.

DAY 123 AFTER SURGERY

Physical therapy – Pelvic Tilt

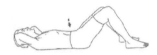

The pelvic tilt is the base for many exercises. When you lie on your back with your knees up and feet flat there is a space between your back and the floor due to the natural curve of the back. During this exercise, you need to flatten your back against the floor by tightening stomach and buttocks muscles.

When you let your breath out, your abdomen should

come towards your back as this happens naturally during exhale. This exercise results in your lower back, gently stretching and reaching in the direction of the floor. Repeat this exercise 30 times per set. Start with one set per session and perform one session per day.

Physical Therapy - Bent Leg Lift

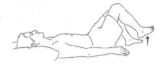

Tighten your stomach to keep your trunk rigid, then slowly raise one leg three or four inches off the floor. Hold this position, and then slowly return to your starting position while keeping your trunk rigid. Repeat with the other leg. Repeat this motion 30 times per set. Do one set per session, and one session per day.

DAY 125 AFTER SURGERY

Physical therapy – Hamstring stretch

Hold your right leg behind the knee on the thigh. If you cannot comfortably reach that position with your hands, you can extend your grip with a towel. Slowly, maintaining your right leg as straight

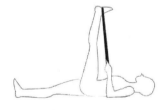

as possible, pull it towards you until you feel the stretch down the back of your thigh.

The goal is to have your leg as perpendicular a possible, but it is more important to keep it straight. So at the beginning the leg might not be vertical, just lift it until you feel a stretch. The stretch is felt in the back of your thigh. By pointing your toes down (towards you) you can further increase the stretch. Hold the stretch for 8-10 seconds and repeat on the other leg. Repeat three to five times per set. Do one set of this exercise per session. Do one to two sessions per day.

Physical therapy – Knee to chest

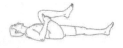

This is a basic exercise that helps to unload your spine. In this position, the pressure on the discs and the joints of the lower back (lumbar spine) are minimal. This exercise helps to decrease the stress on these structures, and it also helps to reduce muscle tension.

To perform this exercise put your hands behind the right knee, pull the knee into the chest until a comfortable stretch is felt in the lower back and buttocks. Keep your back relaxed. Even though the picture shows the other leg stretched out straight, my physical therapist recommended keeping the other knee bent. Repeat this exercise with the left knee.

Repeat this exercise 3-5 times per set, perform one set per session, and complete two sessions per day.

Physical therapy – Lumber Rotation

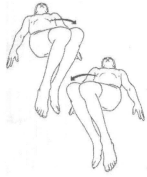

Lie on your back with your knees bent. Keeping your knees together and your shoulders against the floor, roll your knees to one side until you feel a stretch in your back and hip. Slowly rock your knees from side to side in a small, pain-free range of motion. Extend the range as you become more flexible. Hold for 30-60 seconds. Repeat 20 times per set. Do one set per session and one session per day.

DAY 128 AFTER SURGERY

Physical therapy – Bridging

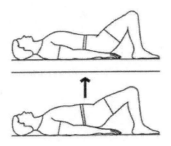

Lay on your back with your knees bent and slowly lift your buttocks from the floor. Keep stomach muscles tightened. Repeat 20 times per set. Do one set per session and one session per day.

DAY 129 AFTER SURGERY

Physical therapy – Extremity Flexion

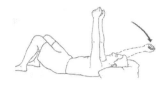

Lying on the floor with your knees bent tighten stomach muscles and slowly lower your right arm to the right side. Then lower your left arm to the left side. If this feels easy, add two-pound weights to each arm.

In the next set of exercises lower your right arm overhead, and then lower your left arm overhead. Keep the arms straight. The longer the leverage, the better the stretch of the back.

Repeat 30 times per set. Perform one set per session and one session per day.

DAY 130 AFTER SURGERY

Physical Therapy – Strengthening Hip Abductor

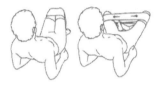

This is a set of two exercises for strengthening. The first one uses a rubber band for resistance, and the second one uses a 10" ball for resistance.

In the first exercise, the band is looped around both legs above the knees. The exercise requires you to tighten stomach muscles and push the knees apart.

The second exercise requires squeezing the ball with

your knees while again tightening stomach muscles.

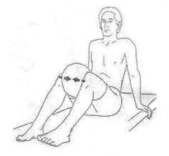

DAY 164 AFTER SURGERY

Kicked out of physical therapy

I have been going to physical therapy twice a week. The physical therapy really helped with flexibility and building general confidence about my back. The therapists had been very creative with their exercises, adding new twists to make old exercises more challenging.

An unfortunate side effect of these exercises was that while my back was getting better my knees were getting worse. Certain movements really made them hurt. The therapists were coming up with exercises to avoid those movements, but they reached the point where they could not give me more exercises without the concern of making my knees worse.

They told me that I need to take a two-week break

to rest my knees. If my knees did not get better, I needed to take care of them before coming back. They gave me guidelines on which exercises I can continue on my own.

DAY 169 AFTER SURGERY

Overall assessment of pain

Overall on day 169, I was doing better, however not back to "normal." I had more flexibility, I was able to pick things up from the floor (if I bend the knees), and I could twist a little to reach for things behind me. I was able lift reasonably heavy grocery bags without pain. I could sit longer, but the leg still got numb if I sat without getting up every hour. My biggest problem was my inability to walk for more than 20-30 minutes without a stop due to pain.

DAY 180 AFTER SURGERY

Back in Physical Therapy

I saw a doctor for the knee pain. The knee problem was tendinitis. He prescribed anti-inflammatory meds, ice three times a day, and physical therapy. The meds and the ice really helped, and my knees began feeling a lot better. I had my PT evaluation for the knees, and we planned on how to continue both the knees and the back rehab at the same time.

Overall assessment of pain

I reached my 6-month anniversary after surgery. I hoped to be feeling better at this point in time. I was not in pain if I did nothing, but any prolonged walking caused pain (some lower back, some around the ankle). If I sat for more than an hour, my leg got numb from the mid-thigh to the ankle.

DAY 275 AFTER SURGERY

No loose screws here!

My nine-month follow-up appointment confirmed that all my screws are in good shape. This was the last appointment with the surgeon.

CONCLUSION

It has been six years since I had my surgery. I think surgery was the right solution for me because it took care of the acute pain I was in for several years; however, the surgery did not return me back to "normal." I am limited in how long I can walk before I am in significant pain. I had to learn what my limitations are, and I can to function normally for the most part.

I hope sharing my experience will help others to be more prepared and know what to expect. I would also appreciate it if you could leave a review on this book as readers depend on each other to locate books with specific and helpful information. I am always interested in hearing from people who want to share their experience. Feel free to reach out and contact me at kadydash@outlook.com.

If you would like to receive a list of all helpful products mentioned in this book with URLs to locate them feel free to email me. You can also find this list on my website: https://kadydash.wordpress.com/2017/07/08/the-list-of-mobility-aids-by-kady-dash.

ALPHABETICAL INDEX

Bedside potty....................3, 21, 23p., 45
Blood pressure...................15, 27, 30, 32
Bowel movement....................16, 23p., 69
Butt Buddy....................4, 6, 27p., 50, 60
Cane................................41p., 53
Catheter........................3, 16, 20p., 32
Celebrex....................6p., 66p., 69, 73p.
Checklist...........................3, 11, 13
Constipation.......................6, 16, 67p.
Disk fusion surgery.........................9
Earplugs..............................26, 42
Grab rail................................51
Grabber ....6, 45, 61p.
Hospital   3p., 9pp., 17pp., 22pp., 29p., 34, 42p., 46, 56
Incision..........18, 23, 34, 38, 48p., 59p., 63pp.
Insurance...................12, 33, 41, 50, 53p.
Long reach bathroom aid.................28, 43
Noise............................16p., 32, 42
Numbness...............................75
Occupational Therapy....................27, 58
Pain med   5p., 11, 16, 23, 25p., 30, 36, 47p.,

55, 57, 59, 65pp.
Phone....................11, 13, 20, 25p., 43, 54
Physical therapy   3, 7p., 18, 27, 37, 52, 58, 65, 77, 79pp., 84pp., 89
Potty...........................3, 21, 23p., 45
Rehab 3pp., 9pp., 19, 23, 25pp., 29pp., 35pp., 40, 42, 44pp., 50pp., 89
Rehabilitation facility   3pp., 9pp., 19, 23, 25, 29, 42, 44, 52, 55pp.
Shampoo hat......................22p., 34, 43p.
Shower.........6, 11, 22p., 34, 43, 51, 59p., 64, 67
Sock buddy............................28p., 46
Spinal fusion surgery..........................9
Sponge bath....................4, 22, 34, 36, 38
Steri-strips...........................6, 59, 67
Surgery   1, 3pp., 14p., 17p., 20, 22pp., 30p., 33pp., 41pp,. 48pp., 52p., 55pp., 60, 62pp., 69pp., 79p., 84pp.
Tens......................4, 33p., 38, 63, 75, 82
Toilet aids...............................25, 43
Unger..................................45, 62
Visiting Nurse....................5p., 52, 56, 70
Walker....................27, 31, 37, 41, 52pp.
Wipe.......................24, 28p., 43, 56, 61
X-ray..............................24, 58, 76

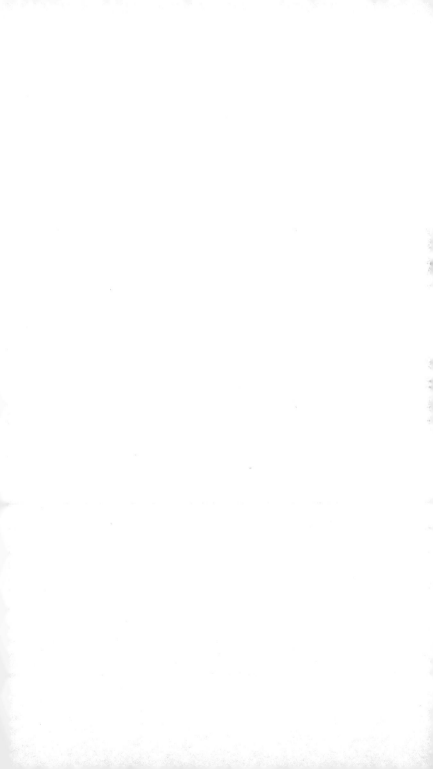

Made in the USA
Monee, IL
02 July 2025